# NEVER RELAPSE INTO WATCHING PORN AGAIN

A DEEP INNER GAME GUIDE TO BUILDING YOUR INNER STRENGTH AND REACHING THE 90-DAYS PORN FREE STREAK

By

**DONNY DRAKO**

I0412356

**Copyright © 2017**

# DISCLAIMER

This book is not intended as a substitute for the medical advice of physicians. The reader should regularly consult a physician in matters relating to his/her health and particularly with respect to any symptoms that may require diagnosis or medical attention.

# TABLE OF CONTENTS

# RECOMMENDED BOOKS

# INTRODUCTION

There is a new revolution going on globally in the lives of men. For the first time in the history of our race, thousands of men are taking an oath of abstinence from masturbation. They are doing this to counter the effects of porn addiction.

The initial target these men set for themselves is to go 90 days without PMO (Porn, Masturbation, and Orgasm). By achieving this target, countless believe that they will achieve superpowers. Some of these superpowers include lack of social anxiety, getting a girl, lack of fear, etc.

But the problem is that, almost 90 % of those who begin, never seem to go beyond the one week mark i.e. they RELAPSE.

Even for the remaining 10 %, it takes a year or two to achieve the 90 days porn free target and become free of their porn addiction.

What is it that makes a select few break free of this porn addiction?

It has taken me at least 10 attempts and close to one and a half years to break the RELAPSE cycle and become free of my addiction. During this time what I realized was that along with the 90 days porn free challenge those who worked on their inner game were the ones who were able to break free.

Before I begin, let me tell you one thing 'Don't believe a word I say'. Now, why would I say that? Because I can only speak from my own experience. None of the concepts, ideas and insights I share are inherently true or false, right or wrong. They simply reflect my own results and the amazing results I have seen coaching other men. Having said that, however, I believe if you apply the techniques in this book you will successfully cross the 90 days porn free streak.

In the first part of the book, I will teach you how to set your long-term goals (purpose or mission) in life. Once you identify your true mission in life, you do not have to be a slave to the external motivational videos or others stories to motivate you. Your own true purpose itself will guide and empower you to achieve the 90 days porn free streak.

In the second part, I will teach you how to replace your porn addiction with a new habit that is also closely linked to your true inner purpose.

In the third part, you will become aware of how the mind tricks you and what you must do in such an emergency, to STOP another RELAPSE.

I have kept this book short and simple. I do not go into the depth of how creating your long term goals or finding your true purpose will transform your LIFE. You can easily get that information within two hours by watching some of the movies like 'Matrix' or Christopher Nolan's 'Batman Begins'.

Use this book as a guide. Take a note of the ideas, skill and techniques you can start working on immediately. Test what works for you and what doesn't. Come back to the book often. Reread the parts as you practice them.

And, this is important, "Don't make the mistake of just reading this book and saying "I know this stuff" before you've mastered the information through your own personal experience.

# CHAPTER 1
# CREATING LONG-TERM GOALS TO BUILD A STRONG INNER FOUNDATION

## FINDING YOUR PURPOSE IN LIFE

Porn Addiction is a sign that you have drifted away from your life's journey and forgotten about it completely. Whatever your life's journey is, you need to find it, and otherwise you would struggle to get out of your addiction for the rest of your life.

Your mind wants a clear, specific and detailed reason to move away from porn. And the reason must be connected to your higher purpose in life.

If, tomorrow you wake up charged with fulfilling your mission in life, all you will care about is the steps you will take to get there. You will be so occupied with your mission that the thought of porn or masturbation wouldn't even run through your mind.

Remember this, 'All POWER is from within and under your control'.

Unless you REALIZE what your true purpose in life is, this POWER would never be revealed to you from within.

It's time for you to know what your true purpose in life is. It's time to get back your INNER POWER.

## HOW TO BECOME CLEAR ABOUT YOUR PURPOSE IN LIFE

There are three simple steps to identifying your goal/purpose/mission in life and practice remembering it in such a way that you never ever forget it in life. The steps are as follows

**STEP 1:** Identify your goal

**STEP 2:** Write it down

**STEP 3:** Remember it and practice writing it down every day when you get up early in the morning.

Before we begin, I want you to get a piece of paper and a pen. Now, as you read further write down your purpose. Write down whatever pops into your mind first. It doesn't have to be clear in the beginning. Just write it down.

**How to Identify Your Purpose?**

Your goal is what you are dissatisfied about the most in life. Ask yourself what are you most frustrated about in your life? What would you like to change?

Ask yourself this important question. 'If you were to live in the world where anything is POSSIBLE, what would you like to achieve?

The next step that I am about to show you will help you become a little bit aware of your goal.

The following is a list of the wants in life. Give a rating from 1 to 10 about how much satisfied you are in that area of life. 1 being completely dissatisfied. 10 being completely satisfied.

1. Girl/Romance

2. Friends and Family

3. Career

4. Money

5. Health

6. Fun and Recreation

e.g. If you haven't had a girlfriend in years because you are shy and introverted and gave a rating of 1 for the first point, then you can put your goal as finding, dating and marrying your soul mate.

There doesn't have to be only one calling in life. There can be many. And all of these callings sometimes do overlap.

Some other questions that you can ask yourself to help you identify your goal

What if you were to die tomorrow? What would you wish you could do before you die?

What would you do if you had unlimited time, money and resources?

What have you always wanted to do, but have not done yet?

What activities or skills do you want to learn or try out?

Another example, in the career section

Goal: End MALARIA in the World.

(By the Way, this is Bill Gates Mission in Life)

Here's what to do right now to create your goal and make sure that you break free of the Relapse cycle.

**BE SPECIFIC**

Your goal must be as clear as possible. E.g. If you write 'I want to be RICH'. Be clear about how rich you want to be. You might write 'i want 1 Million dollars sitting in my bank account by 31$^{st}$ December 2016 so that I could use it to Eradicate AIDS from the face of the Earth.

Being clear about the outcome that you want in life will help you sharpen your inner compass.

Imagine that you live in Toronto. And you want to go on an adventure for a week. If you write down your goal as heading south, you won't reach anywhere, no matter how long you take because anything south of Toronto will make you believe that you have achieved your goal. But making your goal as Sitting on the BEACH AT Rio De Janeiro drinking Virgin Mojito on 31st December. Even if you accidently land up in New Mexico, you will still know where your adventure really is.

## CLEAR AND DETAILED

If you want to go a step further, you can make your purpose as Cristal clear and detailed as possible. E.g. If your goal is '1 Million by Dec 31st, 2016 that I could use to Eradicate Homelessness from the Earth', you can vividly imagine you sitting in your office signing a check of 1 Million to a Charity Foundation or You handling this amount to a contractor who has built 10 thousand homes for the poor.

## FEAR

Choose a purpose that might SCARE you. If it doesn't scare you, then either you are shooting too low or you don't want to believe in yourself. Once you open yourself up to this fear, believing in yourself becomes EASY.

## REMEMBERING AND PRACTICING IT

If you want to reach a 90-day goal of becoming porn free, you just have to avoid relapsing once every day for 90 days. You need to build an inner motivation to fight your ancient primitive instincts. So, it is important to remember your goals daily.

There are two ways to do that.

1. When you get up in the morning, before even brushing your teeth, write down your goal.

2. Find an image that would remind you of your goal. Keep it at a place where you are bound to see it throughout the day.

E.g. If you want to be rich and your mentor is Warren Buffet, You can save an image of him as your Smartphone wallpaper.

# CHAPTER 2
# TAKING THE FIRST STEP: REPLACING YOUR ADDICTION WITH A NEW HABIT

Now, before we begin this chapter, let me tell you this. Don't commit the mistake of comparing your end goal to where you are now and then saying to yourself 'I am only in the mud, it's impossible to land on the moon someday.'. There was a time in your life where you couldn't walk. Now, you can RUN.

If you have found out your mission or at least have a general idea about what it is, then it is time to begin taking Baby Steps towards achieving it.

-**"Take the first step in faith. You don't have to take the whole staircase. Just take the first step"**

**–Dr Martin Luther King Jr**

It's time to begin your journey by taking the baby step, i.e. creating your first habit that is closely aligned with your higher purpose.

You can never replace a habit. You can only change it. Similarly, you can never get out of the habit of watching porn unless you replace it with a new highly productive, purpose driven habit.

So, unless you replace porn with a new habit, the mind will keep on reminding you to watch porn until you RELAPSE again. And you wouldn't like to go back again to the feeling of Pain and the Guilt that comes after you relapse, would you?

## HOW TO CREATE A NEW HABIT

There is a simple three step process to create this new habit. It is given below.

**STEP 1**: Choose a habit that is also connected to your long term goal.

**STEP 2:** Write it down

**STEP 3:** Start doing it NOW.

## EXAMPLES

Let us start with two examples.

**Example 1:**

TRUE PURPOSE: Finding my soul mate

SIMPLE HABIT: Spend 1-hour every day on how to attract a girl. Then, Spend 15 minutes a day talking to girls randomly

**Example 2:**

TRUE PURPOSE: Win the Body-building International Competition

SIMPLE HABIT: SIGN-UP to the Gym and go there every morning at least 4 times a week.

## THINGS TO KEEP IN MIND

Choose a habit that does not require a lot of time in the beginning to do. E.g. If you choose meditation, start with 5 minutes a day.

Also, remember to do it the first thing when you get up in the morning. If you choose another time there is a higher chance that you will procrastinate and not do it. The will power is very high in the morning. So it is better to utilize it for building a highly productive habit.

Create a calendar or buy a new one especially for this new habit. Tick mark it every time you complete the habit. Keep the calendar in such a location that it will also remind you to perform your new habit every time you get up in the morning.

Remember. Be as much specific, clear and detailed as possible, especially for building a new habit.

Another example of a new habit that is clear.

If your purpose is to be the BEST FATHER IN THE WORLD for your 6 year old Daughter. You can start with a habit making it more clear and specific for example 'Help my 6-year-old daughter for 30 minutes every day for completing her homework.

# CHAPTER 3
# IDENTIFYING AND ELIMINATING THE THOUGHTS THAT CAUSE YOU TO RELAPSE

Let's face it. You identify your purpose; create a simple habit to reach that goal. Now, there are still chances that your Brain will try to make you RELAPSE. In fact, the more you try to think long term the bigger will be the resistance put up by the brain.

The mind will make you act like a VICTIM. It might LOWER your self-esteem. Or it might just simply tell you that watching porn is harmless.

Once you give in, you will only realize that you were fooled by your own brain when the GUILT sets in i.e. when you are released from the Matrix of the mind temporarily.

So it is better to identify such thoughts beforehand and be aware when they come, before it's too late.

These thoughts are like the Satan coming every time to give you the Apple. Would you eat it this time as you have eaten it always?

Here are the some of the common thoughts that you need to remember that are mostly likely to trick you into another RELAPSE:

1. 'It's just been two days, you can always start over'

2. 'You will fail eventually, might as well do it now so you can start over'

3. 'All of your friends do it, why resist?'

4. 'It's been 5 days, a little peek won't hurt.'

5. 'It's Sunday. You can masturbate today and tomorrow will be a fresh start. You'll make it to next weekend with ease.'

6. 'Just do it today and then you'll do a long streak.'

Write down at least 3 thoughts that had come into your mind, the last time you had relapsed.

# WHAT TO DO WHEN YOU REALZE THAT YOU ARE HEADING FOR A RELAPSE

It's important to realize these tricks that the mind is playing with you when you hear the thoughts going around in your mind trying to convince you to relapse.

In such an instant, it is necessary to do something immediately that would break the spell.

Some things that you can do immediately to bring yourself out of the Matrix or the Spell

## 1. Dance.

I'll assume you are alone. No one is around. You can simply shake some weird moves on some weird songs quickly. Also, the mind gets satisfied with at least some movement, if not an orgasm. And you win by not giving in.

So, everyone wins!

## 2. Start Breathing Deeply.

Breathing consciously helps you get out of the sexual temptations by making you focus on your breath. This is the classical technique that Buddhist Monks use at the beginning of meditation to control their mind.

Start by inhaling air to the count of 10 seconds. Then wait for 5 seconds and then exhale out the air for another 10 seconds. And then again wait for 5 seconds. Continue the cycle of inhaling and exhaling for at least 10 times.

## 3. Do pushups

Start with pushups. Keep doing this exercise until all your energy is drained out and you cannot continue further. In the end, you will become so exhausted that the thought of even sitting on the computer and looking at porn will simply feel uninteresting.

## A Word of CAUTION if you RELAPSE

When you RELAPSE, you begin to feel a sense of GUILT for giving in.

Now, I have seen many men trying to overcome this painful feeling by covering it with Over-Confidence. They say to themselves that this time they won't give in. That this time, they would successfully conquer their instincts and reach the 90-days porn free streak.

The problem with over-confidence is that it makes you believe that you will remain in such a super high confidence state forever. So, you DO NOT take the necessary steps to prevent a RELAPSE again.

When I first began helping men with the problem of RELAPSE, many highly confident men started approaching me to help them. I believed that my work would be easy.

But I was wrong! The more confident the men were on their first day after a RELAPSE, more work had to be done on them to get them to achieve the 90-day porn free streak.

So, be cautious when the Over-Confidence sets in a after you RELAPSE. Take the necessary steps given in this book, so that you NEVER RELAPSE INTO WATCHING PORN AGAIN!

# CHAPTER 4
# ACCEPT YOUR CALLING

Addiction to Porn is a sign that something somewhere is seriously wrong. Your life is not aligned and it has drifted from its path.

Joseph Campbell in his book The Hero with a Thousand Faces talks about the common story or the myth that each of us follow in our mind. This story is like a blueprint that guides us through our lives and helps us achieve what we want. If we do not follow our own personal story or myth, we usually divert from our own hero's journey and end up with an addiction.

The story follows the following simple steps.

## 1. CALL FOR ADVENTURE

The hero is presented with a call to adventure. He accepts it, leaves his village (comfort zone) and moves towards achieving his true purpose in life

## 2. CONQUERING THE QUEST

Along his journey he faces a lot of trial and tribulations. He, after failing a number of times finally succeeds in achieving his purpose.

## 3. SHARE THE WISDOM

He returns back to where he belonged and shares his wisdom and insight with others around.

If the hero refuses the call, this is what happens.

## 1. REFUSAL OF THE CALL

The hero is too afraid to conquer his fears. Under the pressure to conform, he follows the journey that the society has decided for him.

## 2. FALL INTO THE WASTELAND

His life becomes boring and devoid of any meaning. His soul feels empty. He tries to fill his emptiness through porn or any other addiction.

## 3. ACCEPT OR DIE

This goes on until he accepts his call or he DIES.

Almost all men in the world are stuck up in the first stage of their journey. They refuse to accept their calling and delay it for the rest of their life.  Under the society's pressure to conform, they try to suppress it and bury it in their unconscious. This makes their life boring, dull and miserable.  The 'Call' tries to haunt the man again and again, reminding him of the path that he must take and not the one that the society has decided for him. He refuses it more by falling into addiction and becoming numb to his feelings. This continues for a few years until the pain of denial becomes so high that he fall into the wasteland (e.g. mid-life crisis or depression). The only way to come out of this wasteland is to find and become aware of the deeply buried 'Calling' hidden in the unconscious.

Unless you accept your call for adventure, the mind will keep you in the mode of RELAPSE.

To identify and uncover the ways in which you can become aware of your calling, you can either use the techniques discussed in Part  One of this back or go back into the memory lane of your past and analyze the instances when you refused the call.

Some questions that can help you out.

When you were small what did you think of becoming?

What habits in the past made you truly feel alive?

If you were free to do anything in this world what would you do?

What problem do you find in this world that you believe you can change it?

The mind is a BIG mystery. It won't reveal your purpose completely in the beginning. It will only give you hints and allow you to solve the puzzle on your own. What is important is to accept the calling no matter how wage it is or else keep searching for it as Apple founder Steve Jobs once said

**"The only way to do great work is to love what you do. If you haven't found it yet, KEEP LOOKING. Don't settle. As with all matters of the heart, you'll know when you find it. And, like any great relationship, it just gets better and better as the years roll on. So keep looking until you find it. Don't settle..."**

E.g., Mickey likes mixing music. So at first he accepts his call and move towards become a DJ. Then, after few month or years, he realizes that using an instrument like a violin to create music is much more adventurous and fulfilling. Therefore, he begins his journey to mastery violin. Then, after a couple of years he finds that teaching children violin is much more adventurous and so on goes his story.

Now imagine Mickey instead of becoming a DJ, under the pressure of his father and his teachers studies management and lands up a corporate job that he is not interested in doing. He continues his lifeless, boring, sad and lonely journey for the rest of his life. To counter the boredom and hollowness in his life he falls into addiction and never recovers again.

At the end of his life, when he is about to Die, do you think he would look at his life and say it was full of adventure and taking a corporate job or refusing to become a DJ was the best decision of his life? Imagine the consequences of refusing the 'Call' to him, his family and the world.

Addiction is an effect of a far bigger cause. It acts as a temporary solution to fill your soul that has become empty. Your soul wants a life of meaning and purpose and unless you give it that, it would continue to fill itself through porn.

So, find out what you're 'CALLING' or 'PURPOSE' in life is. Accept it and then begin the journey towards achieving it. You can use Chapter 2 in this book to identify the habits that you can start forming right away to start your journey towards achieving your purpose in Life.

# CHAPTER 5
# THE DEATH GROUND TECHNIQUE

In his book "The 33 STRATEGIES OF WAR" Robert Greene talks about a strategy, he calls it 'THE DEATH-GROUND STRATEGY' He says, you must put yourself in such a situation that the only option left for you is to FIGHT. The only other option being DEATH itself. Under such a situation of urgency, you are sure to succeed.

In ancient times, when leaders went to war and landed on enemy territory, the first thing that they did was burn down the boats that they had used to land there. With no other way left to return back home, this put them and their army with only one choice and that was to WIN. With only this option in hand, the army would become twice or thrice as powerful and fight the enemy with fury, often winning the battle successfully especially when the odds were stacked against them.

The reason that you relapse is that you have many options. You have a thousand options to relapse a thousand times in the future. Every time there is an inner voice that tells you 'I'll watch porn or masturbate only this time. NEXT TIME I'll be serious and not watch porn again'

It is because the mind always has the option of a 'NEXT TIME', it always chooses this choice.

Put yourself in a situation where the only option for you and your mind is to not watch porn again. Leave yourself no room to procrastinate.

When you give yourself only one option and that is to FIGHT the battle of Porn Addiction, you suddenly become ALIVE and reaching 90 days porn free streak becomes easy.

How would you put yourself in such a situation where looking at porn would be equivalent to DEATH or extreme amount of PAIN?

Imagine, you were forced to give $10 to your enemy. Would you feel the pain? How about $100 or $1000? Do you feel the pain now? Is it bigger than the pain of going back to watch porn again? If it is then try this technique step by step as follows.

**STEP 1:** Decide the amount you would feel extremely painful to give to your enemy.

**STEP 2:** Suppose you choose $100. Give three times the money i.e. $300 to a close friend of yours who you TRUST.

**STEP 3:** Tell your friend to be accountable to you by giving your enemy $100 each time you RELAPSE.

**STEP 4:** If you do not fail or fail at least once, which I am sure, you will not, then take back the remaining money from your friend at the end of 90 days.

Your brain is super amazing when it comes to calculating PAIN. It sees PAIN as DEATH. When you are about to relapse, it will automatically calculate watching porn once equal to loosing $100 and the pain of giving it to your enemy is equal to the pain being unbearable. Your mind will prevent itself from watching Porn because now you have linked it to a deep Irrational pain instead of pleasure.

Before, your mind ran towards Porn for PLEASURE. Now it will run against it to avoid the PAIN.

Be sure to tell your friend to give the money to your enemy after you RELAPSE, even if you tell him not to later. You will feel the REAL pain for the first time that you RELAPSE. This will motivate your mind not to watch Porn even more the next time.

If you have no enemy, then tell your friend to donate it to the Political party you hate the most. If you are, a Republican then tell your friend to donate it to The Democratic Party or vice versa.

Another variation that you can try is using EMBARASSMENT to your own advantage. To your mind EMBARASSMENT = DEATH.

What secret of yours would you like the people around you not to know? Will you be willing to pay $100 to the person who is blackmailing you into releasing your secret to the public?

You can apply this technique step-by-step as follows

**STEP 1:** Tell your closest friend THREE secrets about you that you want no one to know about.

Here is an Example of a secret. "I was slapped once by a girl' 'I was robbed by a 13 year old girl once' ' I was called Monkey when I was small.'

Choose a secret about you that no one know about and the very thought of which makes you feel uncomfortable.

**STEP 2:** If you RELAPSE then, tell your friend to release one of the secrets to at least 5 people that you know and hate. Alternatively, best, release it on Facebook.

If your friend does not want to look bad, then tell him to send an email to them through an anonymous account.

So, would your mind be READY to allow other people to know your secret in exchange for watching porn?

If the answer is NO, then Go Forward with this technique and you sure will achieve the Porn Free 90 day challenge with ease.

# RECOMMENDED BOOKS

If you want help with

1. Finding your true purpose/passion/mission in life

-Man's Search For Meaning – Viktor Frankl

-Drive: The Surprising Truth About What Motivates Us by Daniel H. Pink

-Start with Why: How Great Leaders Inspire Everyone to Take Action- Simon Sinek


2. Creating and maintaining a new Habit

-Willpower: Rediscovering the Greatest Human Strength by Roy F. Baumeister

-The Power of Habit: Why We Do What We Do in Life and Business by Charles Duhigg

# FREE BONUS

If you would like to be guided step by step for the first 90 days and want me to be accountable to you, send me an E-mail at DrakoDonny@gmail.com

P.S. This offer is limited only to the first 20 people who contact me directly.

# CAN I ASK A FAVOUR?

If you enjoyed this book, found it useful or otherwise, then I'd really appreciate it if you would post a short review on Amazon. I do read all the reviews personally so that I can continually write what people are wanting.

If you'd like to leave a review then please visit the link below:

(http://www.amazon.com/gp/product/B016FSFC5I)

Thanks for your support!